Title:

Making her scream and moan.

Give her a breathtaking and passionate foreplay that will leave her asking for more of you.

By

Loveth sherly

Table of content

doesn't for the woman in your life.

- Seduction is an act of arousing her
- You can take her body if you seduce her mind.
- How to Seduce a Woman in Bed
- Touch her at every opportunity, but be subtle about it.
- Make your touch more personal and sensuous, rather than bold and fun.
- Increasing the sexual tension by kissing her.

10. <u>Anal is not homosexual.</u>
11. <u>Fantasy is typical.</u>
12. <u>Threesomes for oral sex</u>

Introduction

This book is intended to provide reliable information on how to make her scream and moan in complete delight. You will learn how to satisfy a woman by increasing the intensity of your sexual games. Some men feel that the amount of thrust they can execute during intercourse makes them superhuman.

Sex is much more than simply hitting her clitoris and hammering her with your rod penis.

Few things can make a girl moan and scream like working on her erogenous zones; thus, learning this technique on her erogenous zones is essential. (FOREPLAY)

Many guys, however, make the mistake of making sex only about them. This merely limits the range of emotions you may send to her through passionate sex, which is considerably more than penetrative sex.

It is much more important for women to engage their emotions and minds while also paying attention to all of their physical parts.

The majority of men prefer it when a woman is very talkative during sex. And this book guarantees to assist you in doing so.

Chapter 1

The great arousal

For most guys, satisfying a lady is a daunting task. Understanding what makes her tick and what sorts of strokes and touches she likes may appear difficult, but rest assured, you can learn how to please her hotspots and guarantee she has a good time every time.

Pleasing a lady in the bedroom isn't as difficult as it appears, and having the desire to do so is a significant part of the struggle.

What are the symptoms of a woman being aroused?

How long does a lady take to become aroused?
Is there anything I can do to arouse her?
So, if you're interested in making her experience

enjoyable, you're already halfway there.

To be amazing in bed with a lady , you must first understand her body and the trigger points that get her on.

That being said, it is occasionally necessary to have a bit more knowledge and know-how than you may assume.

Let's speak about how important it is to understand female arousal triggers and how to completely excite a lady so she wants more.

You can try these tips to increase her arousal tonight.

If you want to increase your partner's arousal and sexual desire, you've come to the right spot.

Arousal Differences Between Males and Females

You've undoubtedly heard that men and women get aroused differently in general.

Men and women have significant physical and mental

variations in how they perceive arousal.

It is natural for male and female arousal patterns to differ because of variances in the male and female brains.

This is because the sex-steroid hormones that pass through our bodies differ across genders.

According to research, hormones in women, primarily estrogen and progesterone, and testosterone in men can alter the sexual experience for either sex.

These hormones have a wide range of effects on brain chemistry. Our socialization also plays a role: males may prefer visual triggers such as watching pornography, while women may prefer to be romanced or to believe that their lover actually sees and desires them.

While watching an X-rated film may be enough to get you in the mood, she may require a romantic date night or plenty of foreplay, such as kissing and touching before she is in the mood.

Recognizing Female Arousal Triggers

Being present and involved is one of the best ways to get your partner in the mood for sex.

Giving your spouse your undivided attention before entering the bedroom, such as putting your phone aside and engaging in a meaningful discussion at the dinner table, can do more to set the scene than simply lighting a few candles.

However, creating the mood is equally vital.

It is recommended that males engage in some 'chore play,' that is, helping to clean up the house and doing their share of chores, so that she has more time to rest and practice self-care.

The better she looks after herself, the more attractive she will feel, and the more ready she will be for intimacy.

Tips to Turn Her On How to Arouse a Woman

Men are sometimes compared to microwaves during sex because they are ready to go in an instant.

Women, on the other hand, are like crockpots in that they take longer to heat up.

This leads us to our first point.

1. Don't be hasty.

Remember that your mate is a slow cooker.

So, if you want to have intimacy later that night, attempt to establish the tone all day. You may:

Send her enticing and flirtatious text messages.

Congratulate her on her beautiful clothing.

So she can practice yoga, she should do the dishes.

On the couch, pour yourself a glass of wine.

Create the easygoing, seductive energy she craves.

If your girlfriend isn't in the mood for intimacy, there are alternative methods to connect with her physically:

Make an offer to draw her a bubble bath.

Provide her with a massage.

Snuggle up on the couch with her and watch a movie.

Find tactile methods to interact with her, such as holding her hand or caressing her hair.

This will make her feel more linked and calm, which may lead to increased desire in the future.

2. Set the stage.

Women enjoy being turned on in the appropriate environment. This includes her favorite candles, soft lighting, and a little romantic music.

All of these elements in your house, when combined, might elicit emotions of sexual desire.

Setting the environment for her demonstrates that you care about her feeling at ease and wanted. Of course, you're going to be admiring her beautiful figure while you're having foreplay.

3. Maintain eye contact.

Don't forget to make lots of direct eye contact with her. Many women want that immediate connection; therefore, this is a great turn-on for them. This simple deed has the power to make women feel worshiped and desired.

4. Tell her how hot she is.

Don't be afraid to compliment her on her beauty and sexiness. This can boost her confidence in the bedroom, allowing her to appreciate the sexual moments you share with her more.

You may also utilize this opportunity to have emotionally charged conversations with her. Tell her everything you want to do to her and everything you want her to do to you.

5. Make use of foreplay.

Foreplay is an extremely crucial aspect of sex. The body

of a woman needs time to respond to touch and friction. If you feel like you're becoming aroused too quickly and may climax too soon, it's definitely a good time to try to postpone ejaculation using a doctor-created spray that may take your bedroom play to the next level.

6. Discover Her Erogenous Zones

Erogenous zones are extra-sensitive areas of the body that react to sexual stimulation.

So, it's not only her vulva (the outside part of the female vagina) and clitoris (which are placed inside the labia majora toward the top of her labia minora, or inner labia).
You must also pay attention to other parts of her body.
Her erogenous zones include:
Ears
Her neck at the nape
Wrist inside
Fingertips
Backside
Scalp
Armpits
The lower back

Stomach
Her knees are at the back.

To find out what gets her eager for more, use a combination of soft kisses, leisurely strokes, and gentle massaging on these distinct areas.

7. Generously provide oral pleasure

Don't be afraid to orally gratify her. This is perhaps the finest approach to inducing orgasm in a woman during sex.
Not all women have orgasms just through intercourse.

8. Take Note of Her Cues

Woman lying down, massaging her breasts while excited

Her body will naturally notify you that you're on the correct track.

Look for female arousal signals or indicators like hers:

Dilated pupils
Her back was arched.

Nipples are becoming brittle.
Flushing of the face
Her natural lubricant is heating up.
All of these are solid signals that you're making her want to have sex with you.

9. Show self-assurance.

Confidence is a significant turn-on.

If you exude confident and secure energy, it will make your partner feel desired and will instill sexual confidence in her as well.

So be daring.

10. Allow yourself to be vulnerable.

 Be your most authentic self. Strut your thing, and remember that confidence goes a long way toward having sexual enjoyment in the bedroom.

11. Generously provide oral pleasure

Don't be afraid to orally gratify her. This is perhaps the finest approach to inducing orgasm in a woman during sex.

Not all women have orgasms just through intercourse.

A graph demonstrates that penetrative sex alone does not fully excite most women.

When it comes to reproduction, women are more likely to have an orgasm when they are "engaged in a variety of sexual acts, including oral sex."

Men, on the other hand, are more likely to have orgasms from intercourse alone.

Learn some exciting new oral methods, like using your hands as well as your mouth, and remember to vary your pressure.

You'll be able to tell if she's opening up to you and appreciating your technique with your fingers.
If you're not completely sure in this area, it's time to work on it.
It also doesn't hurt to tell her how much you like doing it.
Some women are scared that their man may not like oral sex, which reduces their enjoyment and relaxation during the act.

Showing your girlfriend that you actually like going down on her can make her enjoy it even more.

Takeaways

Having excellent sex with the one you love on a regular basis is typically a work in progress.

Experimenting with these ideas and tactics to discover what arouses your spouse in bed can only lead to better sex in the long run.

You'll rapidly discover what works and what doesn't for the woman in your life.

The more invested you are in her enjoyment, the more pleasure you will undoubtedly receive in return.

Sexual arousal (also known as sexual excitement) refers to the physiological and psychological reactions that occur prior to or during sexual intercourse. A variety of physiological responses occur in the body and mind in preparation for sexual intercourse, and these responses persist during intercourse. Male excitement results in an **erection**, but female arousal results in engorged sexual tissues such as the **nipples, vulva, clitoris, vaginal walls, and vaginal** lubrication.

Sexual arousal may be influenced by both mental and physical inputs, such as touch and internal hormonal fluctuations. Beyond the mental excitement and the physiological changes that accompany it, sexual arousal has multiple phases and may not result in any actual sexual action. Sexual arousal peaks during an orgasm when there is enough sexual stimulation. Even in the absence of an orgasm, it can be pursued for its own sake.

A person might be sexually stimulated by a multitude of causes, both physical and mental, depending on the context. A person can be sexually aroused by another person, certain qualities of that person, or a non-human item. Physical stimulation of an erogenous zone or acts of foreplay can cause arousal, especially when combined with the prospect of impending sexual action. A romantic setting, music, or other relaxing circumstances can all help to increase sexual excitement. Porn or other sexual media can cause sexual desire. Potential sexual arousal cues differ from person to person and from period to period, as does the amount of arousal.

Stimuli are grouped into three types based on the

sense   involved:
somatosensory (touch), visual, and olfactory (scent). Conversation, reading, films or images, or a smell or setting are all examples of erotic stimuli that can result in sexual arousal. Given the correct circumstances, they may result in the person desiring physical touch, such as kissing, cuddling, and petting an erogenous zone. This may lead to a desire for direct sexual stimulation of the breasts, nipples,pussy, buttocks, and/or

genitals, as well as more sexual activity.

Erotic sensations may come from sources unrelated to the target of later sexual attraction. Many people, for example, may find nudity, erotica, or pornography sexually arousing. This may result in a general sexual desire that is fulfilled by sexual action. Sexual fetishism, or paraphilia, is a condition in which sexual pleasure is obtained or is dependent on the usage of items.

Women, it is commonly assumed, take longer to achieve arousal. However, a recent scientific study has revealed that there is no significant difference in the time it takes men and women to become completely aroused. thermal imaging to capture baseline temperature changes in the vaginal region in order to determine the time required for sexual arousal. Researchers analyzed the time necessary for an individual to achieve the peak of sexual arousal when watching sexually explicit videos or photographs and discovered that women and men took almost the same amount of time to reach the top of sexual excitation around 10 minutes. The amount of time required for foreplay is unique and varies based on the situation.

Humans, unlike many other species, do not have a mating season, and both sexes are theoretically capable of sexual excitement all year.

Seduction is an act of arousing her

Knowing what she truly wants and progressively offering it to her in a way that takes her breath away is the art of seduction. not known

Negatively, seduction entails using temptation and enticement, frequently sexual in nature, to lead someone astray into making a behavioral decision they would not have made if they were not in a state of sexual arousal.

Seduction, when viewed positively, is a synonym for the act of charming someone male or female through an appeal to the senses, often with the goal of reducing unfounded fears and leading to their "sexual emancipation." Some sides in contemporary academic debate contend that the morality of seduction is determined by the long-term effects on the individuals involved rather than the act itself and may not necessarily carry the negative connotations expressed in dictionary definitions.

You can take her body if you seduce her mind.

Being a master of seduction entails generating harmony by pleasing every area of her mind so that she feels at ease in your presence.

And if you can charm her head, you'll be able to seduce her body as well.

A female wants to feel unique, and she wants to see that you're trying. And, sure, you

will notice several signals that she is putting you to the test.
When it comes to wooing women, this is sound advice: if you can make her feel unique, you've accomplished half of your task.

Remember, it's all in their heads; if you can make her feel like a goddess, she'll feel seduced, and if she feels that way, she'll behave that way, too.

The secret to success is to make her feel seduced rather than simply enticing her.

And, in order to make her feel seduced, you must work on yourself, be persistent, and, most importantly, be patient.

Never, ever hurry!

If you hurry things, it will have a negative impact, and the damage will be nearly permanent. Instead, take things carefully and respond in accordance with her body language.

How to Seduce a Woman in Bed

There is no greater thrill than meeting a girl and luring her from the restaurant to the bedroom. Although you know how to seduce a girl via text messages, luring her onto the bed differs from text messages. In this section, you will have insights into how to seduce a girl for sex.

1. Create the ideal environment.

It's time to increase your game now that she's at ease in your company; creating a romantic atmosphere is the first step in wooing her.

2. Experiment with music

You can improve her mood with music but make sure you know her musical preferences as well. Choose a style of music she enjoys, but also slow, calming, and seductive tracks. Try playing some slower music from a band she enjoys. Experts recommend using gentle music to generate a sexual mood, which could be an excellent starting point for attracting a woman.

3. Remember the fragrance's role

Want to know how to seduce a girl when you meet her? Use your olfactory sense. A pleasing fragrance is essential to successfully seducing a woman when you invite her around. A light vanilla aroma or sandalwood are good choices for pleasant but not overpowering scents.

4. The Personal Touch

If you want to know how to seduce a girl for sex, keep the touch factor in mind. Get close, but not too close, so she feels your presence, but don't freak her out. Move closer to her at every opportunity, but don't act aggressively. Just be friendly and closer. You only need to let her feel the warmth of your body; the rest is up to her imagination.

5. Begin getting intimate.

Make the first move gently, sitting close and touching her

knee or shoulder to begin. Again, pace is important in seduction, and going too quickly can turn women off. The first kiss should be soft, longer than a peck, but not a full-on embrace. Make her yearn for more.

6. Locate her erogenous spots

Another way to seduce a girl physically is through erogenous zones. Erogenous zones are body areas that can arouse sexual desire when touched, kissed, licked, or otherwise caressed. Although everyone has different erogenous zones, many women appear to have sensitive skin in specific places on their bodies, and as a result, they may enjoy being kissed, sucked on, licked, and lightly bit.

7. Move slowly.

The key to seduction is to keep the momentum flowing. Moving too rapidly might make someone feel uneasy or turn them off, so take it slowly as you move ahead and understand her goals so you can both enjoy it.

Begin slowly and steadily.

Before you can learn how to captivate women with your touch, you must first understand how to use your body physically appropriately.

So the secret to contacting her is to begin slowly and steadily, gradually increasing the strength of your touch.

Touch her at every opportunity, but be subtle about it.

When you greet her, shake her hand or give her a short embrace, and then while you're talking to her and making a point, softly touch her arm to underline what you're saying. Hold her hand as you cross the street, and when you enter a building or climb into a car, place your hand on her lower back to lead her in.

Give her a high-five whenever she says something amusing or cool, and when you tell her a story about other people touching, illustrate it to her by touching her as well.

After a while, you can take her hand in yours and walk her around the date.

You'll eventually start flirting and joking, and your touch will become much more daring than previously.

When teasing or kidding around, you can embrace her, lift her up and spin her around, bump her hip, tickle her, or shove her on the side. I like to playfully wrap my arms around women and shake them a little.

All of this will gradually make women feel more at ease with you and your physique so that when you take more personal actions, she will already be accustomed to your touch.

Here's how to charm a woman with touch correctly.

You're ready to learn about the strategies now that you know how to make women used to you touching them.

These are methods of touching women to create sexual tension, causing the ladies you touch to become aroused and begin thinking wicked thoughts about you, causing them to want to be more personal with you, accept your advances, and take things further.

You should be quite comfortable with each other at this time; after all, you've been flirting and groping her at every chance.
You've finished flirting with her, so now it's time to attract a lady with a touch.

Make your touch more personal and sensuous, rather than bold and fun.

- Take her hand and play with it while you're talking about something, then gently massage her palm and fingers to show her that you know how to give her pleasure. After a while, run your finger up her arm to her elbow, which will send shivers down her spine, and she might even touch your chest.

- At this point, you can also touch her neck and shoulders. For example, if you want to whisper something in her ear, get closer to her, put your fingers behind her neck, and lean in. After you whisper something sensual in her ear, like how beautiful she is, you can try leaving your hand on her shoulder and continue talking like that.

- Put your arm around her and enjoy the moment as she grows accustomed to your proximity.

- The longer you have your arm over her, the better, and you may even give her a good shoulder or neck rub if she's only been sending you positive signs.
- Feel her face and hair to check whether she likes you.
- After you've gotten to know her, you'll want to know if she's ready to be kissed, which you can simply determine by stroking her hair and face.

When a woman allows you to touch her above the neck, it shows she trusts you sufficiently and is comfortable with you being that close; similarly, if she responds to you stroking her hair or face, you'll quickly know where you stand with her.

Simply by remarking on her hair in any way, such as "your hair looks really soft," you may generate an excellent chance to touch it. Then reach out to touch it and observe her reaction.

There are also numerous ways you can touch her face. One cheesy yet effective way is to gesture that she has a bit of sauce in the corner of her mouth. When she tries to wipe it off, reach out and wipe it off for her with your thumb, keeping your hand close to her face as you give her a knowing smile

If she pulls away or swipes your hand away, it suggests she still doesn't trust you and isn't comfortable enough with you to let you touch her like that; if she reacts positively, it means she genuinely likes you.

Again, observe her reaction and see what she does; if everything goes well and she enjoys it, you may begin making more personal gestures.

Increasing the sexual tension by kissing her.

She'll be incredibly drawn to you if you've done everything perfectly up to this point.
This is the ideal time to charm her by inciting high sexual tension with your touch.
You can do this in a variety of ways, but my favorite is to sit and bring her closer so she sits on top of me, allowing our

faces to be near and my arms to be free to hug her and run my fingers up her thighs before pulling her in to make out with her.

Another effective and straightforward method to make your move is to just place your hand on the back of her head and draw her in close to you, but don't kiss her yet. Hold this posture so your faces are barely inches apart, and it seems like you want to kiss her but tease her about it.

Say something sexual to her and maintain continuous eye contact while holding her head with your hand; you may also softly massage her scalp with your fingertips to give her nice shivers.

She'll eventually melt from the sexual tension, and then you may move in for the kiss.

Going for more than just a kiss

A third approach to entice her with touch is to pin her against a wall, sofa, or bed, which is a fairly forceful gesture that some women adore, and then begin teasing her with kisses.

Kiss her on the neck, shoulders, and wherever else you can except the lips at this moment, since this will increase her excitement and anticipation.

When you believe you've tormented her enough, go in for that passionate kiss she's been waiting for; she won't be able to resist. If you're in a secluded place, you may start taking her clothing off.

So you now know how to charm a lady with a touch in a way that will make her desire you.

Remember not to hesitate while caressing a lady, since hesitation and uncertainty will make her think you're frightened and unsure of yourself. Keep your actions calm, steady, and purposeful, and you'll go far.

Chapter 2

FOREPLAY EXPERTISE

Any sexual action before intercourse is referred to as foreplay. If you don't want it, penetrative sex doesn't have to be the grand finale or even on the menu. When done effectively, great foreplay is plenty hot. Foreplay actually gets the juices flowing by raising sexual arousal—not sexual desire, though it can accomplish that as well.

Sexual excitement generates a variety of physiological reactions in your body, including increased heart rate, pulse rate, and blood pressure; blood vessel dilatation, including genital dilation, which increases blood flow to the genitals, causing swelling of the labia, clitoris, and penis; breast swelling and erect nipples; and vaginal lubrication, which can make intercourse more comfortable and avoid discomfort. Yes, foreplay is pleasurable, but it goes deeper than that. Foreplay promotes emotional connection, which may make you and your spouse feel more connected in and out of the bedroom. And if stress has dampened your libido, a little foreplay may help. Kissing, for example, causes oxytocin, dopamine, and serotonin to be released. This chemical combination reduces cortisol levels (the stress hormone) while increasing emotions of attachment, connection, and happiness. First and foremost: To various folks, foreplay entails different things.

Foreplay in sex is typically characterized as sexual stimulation preceding penetration. If intercourse is excluded, foreplay is defined as an action or behavior that occurs before an event. That "event" may not appear the same to you as it does to someone else, and that's just OK. It does not have to result in intercourse. Intercourse does not have to be the major "course" or even on the menu if it is not desired. It may even be the main event!

Foreplay can stand on its own and be sufficient to achieve orgasm. In reality, research has long demonstrated that many people with vaginas do not orgasm only through intercourse. As a result, as long as there is agreement, foreplay may be and contain whatever you desire. You may even begin before the temperature rises. You have to start somewhere, don't you? But who says you have to be in the thick of things or even in the same room to get started?

If you know you'll be coming together later that day or in a few days, you may utilize foreplay to start and keep the celebration going. Here are a few ideas to get you started. Make a note of it. You don't even have to be inventive to get them started with a note! A message placed in their gym bag or left on their pillow implying that they can't wait to get down and dirty later should do the trick.

1.Send her a text.

Texting is simple and can be done on the go. A fast text telling them what you're going to do to them or how hot you get when they [fill in the gaps] is guaranteed to get things moving south of the border. It also lets them know you're thinking about them, which everyone appreciates. Get together for supper or drinks. Footsies beneath the table, a brief make-out session in the toilet or parking lot, or a cheeky glimpse at what you're wearing or not wearing beneath your clothing. These are just a few ideas for transforming a pre-fun dinner or drink into foreplay. Setting the Mood:

2. Creating the Ideal Environment

Foreplay Setting the tone is a crucial part of perfecting foreplay. Lighting, music, and fragrance may all contribute to a sense of closeness and sensuality. A calm, romantic mood may be created with soft, low lighting and a soothing soundtrack. Experiment with different aromas, such as candles or incense, to create a seductive atmosphere. Don't forget to consider the actual surroundings, such as the temperature and the comfort of the bed or sofa.

3. Communication is another key component of preparing for foreplay.

Talk to your partner about what they enjoy and dislike. Inquire about their desires and dreams. This allows you to adjust the environment to their preferences, making the encounter more pleasurable for both of you. Finally, consider introducing some sensual touch into the environment. The tactile sensation may be enhanced by soft blankets, silky sheets, and plush pillows. Massage oils or lotions can also be used to improve the feeling of touch. Remember that the idea is to create a pleasant, calm, and intimate setting.

3. **Kiss with sincerity**

Send them out or greet them with a kiss. Instead, lock your gaze on them, press your body against them, and give them a long and deep kiss. Make use of your tongue and your hands, and moan just enough to get them excited about what's to come. One of the most intimate and sensuous components of foreplay is kissing. It can aid in the development of a deeper connection between couples as well as the creation of a sense of comfort and security. A good kiss involves more than just the lips; it also involves the tongue, hands, and the entire body. Experiment with various kisses, such as gentle pecks, intense lip locks, and nibbling on the lips and ears. Remember that kissing should be fun and reciprocal, so don't be shy about taking turns or asking for what you want. Kissing has also been demonstrated to have several health advantages. It can strengthen your immune system by exchanging microorganisms and generating antibodies, as well as produce endorphins, which relieve stress and promote sensations of pleasure. Kissing can also benefit your oral health by boosting saliva production, which aids in the removal of dangerous germs and the prevention of tooth decay. Kissing is thus not just a pleasurable and intimate action, but it may also be beneficial to your general health. Provide her with a "thigh job." "Use your fingers, palms, tongue, toys, and lips to slither, lick, and kiss all around their inner thighs

without diving in between their legs," "Hover your mouth over their lips and clit to build desire, and make them ache for more." Investigate their whole body. Don't only focus on your partner's genitals. **Erogenous zones on the body**
 include the neck, thighs, and breasts. "Genitals are fascinating and fun, but try to spend some time focusing on your partner's entire body instead of going straight for her crotch. "Try caressing, licking, or nibbling other erogenous zones, such as her

neck, back, ears, belly, or wrists.

Different Strokes for Different People:

Making Foreplay to Her Preferences Keep in mind that every woman is unique, and what works for one may not work for another. It is critical to tailor foreplay to your partner's tastes in order to create a gratifying and joyful encounter. Request feedback and make changes as needed. If your lover prefers a gentler touch, concentrate on light caresses and teasing strokes. Include nasty banter in your routine if she responds positively to it. The more you know about your partner's likes and dislikes, the more you will be able to personalize the experience to her tastes. It's also crucial to remember that preferences might shift over time. What worked in the past for your spouse may not work as well now.

Communication is essential in any sexual connection, so check in with your spouse on a regular basis and ask if they have any new interests or preferences they'd like to explore. Remember that the aim is for both people to have a joyful and gratifying experience, so don't be hesitant to try new things and explore together.

Locate the clitoris

The key to vaginal and vulval fingering is to identify the clitoris (which is positioned outside the vaginal opening). 'Using only one finger, feel fleshy folds of skin on either side of your vagina below the clit. 'This is the labia. Once you've mastered the anatomy, avoid going straight for the clitoris. This may be quite sensitive, and most individuals will want some preparation before having their clit handled. 'Begin by softly dragging one or two fingers over the labia. Most individuals will notice that when they massage their labia, they begin to grow moist if they are already turned on. This moisture will function as a lubricant for more fingering.'

Using Props and Toys to Enhance Foreplay Props and Toys may be an enjoyable and effective method to improve foreplay. Vibrators, massage oils, and blindfolds can all be utilized to intensify and sensualize the encounter. Tease and tantalize using props such as feathers, ice cubes, or silk scarves. Remember that communication is essential when adding props and toys into the bedroom.

Before you start, make sure you are both comfortable and excited.

It is critical to keep safety in mind when employing props and toys. Before utilizing any toys or props, make sure they are clean and in good shape. To avoid discomfort or irritation, use a water-based lubrication when using a vibrator. Additionally, if restraints are used, ensure that they are not overly tight and can be quickly removed in the event of an emergency. Experimenting with different props and toys may also assist in keeping things interesting in the bedroom and prevent boredom. Experiment with various textures, temperatures, and feelings to determine what works best for you and your partner. And don't be scared to experiment with new things every now and again!

Passionately devouring (Eating) her pussy

The clitoris contains around 8,000 nerve endings! so don't push yourself too much. You may also begin with indirect stimulation by licking in circles around the clitoris. When it comes to stroking and licking, clitorises and vulvas typically demand varying degrees of hardness, so pay attention to your partner's verbal and physical indications. Begin with a gentle kiss from her mouth to her breasts. Continue kissing her body as you approach her waist and hips. Place a hand on either leg and slowly widen it as you approach her underpants. Erogenous zones are areas that are highly sensitive and get a lady on and you might be shocked by some of them! Don't bother with pulling off her pants just yet. Instead, kiss her vulva or vagina through her pants and perhaps softly squeeze it with your lips. You may also gently run your tongue over her vagina from bottom to clitoral.

After kissing her through her underwear for a few minutes, move your kisses slightly lower along her inner thigh. You may go all the way down to the inside of her knee here, but the more you get away from her vagina, the less sensitive it becomes. Kiss her down along her inner thigh with one leg, then back up and switch to the other. If she likes it harsher, gently pinch the flesh of her inner thigh between your lips or perhaps your teeth, but don't be too rough. Otherwise, you run the danger of gravely injuring her. You may even suck the skin here to give her a hickey; only she will see. Spend a bit more time kissing her vagina outside of her underpants while crossing to the other leg. Don't be shocked if she begs you to start eating her out at this point. If she does, try to keep the speed moderate to keep the suspense going. Move your way up her clitoral area to the top of her underwear and put some light kisses on her mons (the area above her clitoris) before removing her underpants.

Taking her panties Off:

If she hasn't already taken them off, place your fingers on either side of her pants, on the outside of her hips, and slowly pull them down until they are completely off. Close Call: Begin slowly kissing and licking (very softly) all around her vagina and clitoral area. As you move around, the edge of your lips should make a little bit of contact with her vagina and clitter, constantly tormenting her.

Give her the middle finger.

It's a lot of fun to devour her pussycat with your fingers. It allows you to offer her more stimulation, stimulate her both within and externally, and provide her with a lot of variety. There are several techniques to finger her while eating her out, some of which are simple to execute while others are extremely uncomfortable.

Finger Her G Spot and Lick Her Clit

Licking her clit or adopting the Under Pressure method, which involves exerting extra pressure under her clit while fingering her G Spot, is an excellent way to get your fingers into the mix. Oral and manual sex (fingering), as well as deep kissing, are the three activities most likely to get a woman off. So oral sex abilities may be more crucial than making your penis bigger or staying in bed longer. You may also use your free hand to press down on her mons pubis to externally stimulate the G-spot. Some ladies prefer it when you rub this region.

Suck Her Clit and Finger Her Vaginal

Bottom Keep in mind that the bottom of some women's vaginas is not exceptionally sensitive; however, the bottom of many women's vaginas in the rear is quite sensitive. Unless you have really long fingers, you may have difficulty reaching it. You may always use a penis-shaped vibrator in place of your finger if you have one. "If you go in too hard and fast, you may feel her flinch or yelp, so take it easy!" You may gradually increase the pressure as her arousal increases, but if in doubt, always go lighter first. Make use of the tip of your tongue. Play recommends utilizing the tip of the tongue in your oral game if your spouse prefers more targeted, concentrated pleasure. "The tip of the tongue can apply more targeted pressure and movement, especially once a vulva owner gets more aroused," he said. "Remember to pay attention to your tongue's tactile sensations to ensure you're licking the clit and not just all over the place." This is a more prevalent issue than you may think." Make use of the flat section of your tongue. Some owners of clitoris prefer a more widespread feeling, while others enjoy a mix of focused and broad stimulation. Vulva owners are unquestionably beings of limitless delight. Playing attention with the flat area of your tongue is a warm-up approach for some, but it's the major draw for others! Lick up and down, in circles, and side to side with the tip of your tongue. As you explore, keep your tongue relaxed. While licking your partner's clitoris, use your palm to apply pressure to the remainder of the vulva (this stimulates the whole clitoris) or softly touch just above their pubic mound to apply G-spot stimulation from outside the body. If your spouse appreciates vaginal stimulation, insert one or two fingers inside their vagina. Thrusting, a "come hither" action, or persistent pressure at the front of the vaginal wall may be pleasurable to your partner. You may even insert a finger via the backdoor if your companion is playing. Simply apply lubrication for any internal anal play., which is why you should try to replicate the feeling with your own tongue. And if you want to utilize a sucking sex toy while penetrating with your hands or tongue, go ahead! Remember that sucking to the finish line isn't a certain strategy to make your spouse cum. In truth, there isn't a one-sex strategy that works for everyone. Some people enjoy having their clitoris sucked, while others are ambivalent about it. Pay attention to what your spouse loves and dislikes, and if in doubt, ask them.

Oral sex

like all sex, is a "choose your own adventure" type of thing. Take note of your partner's body language. If your spouse is thrusting their vulva into your face and groaning, you know what you're doing is effective. Try something else if they're pushing away or are silent. Again, if you're unsure whether your technique is what your partner's body requires, ask questions.

Quickies / Long Sessions:

How to Time Your Foreplay Depending on the environment and the desires of both parties, the timing of foreplay might vary. Quickies may be fun and spontaneous, but prolonged encounters can create anticipation and lead to more powerful orgasms. Pay attention to your partner's signals and make adjustments as needed. If she appears to want more, consider extending the foreplay. A shorter session might still be fulfilling if you're short on time or just seeking a fast release. The key is to communicate with your spouse and to be willing to try new things. It's crucial to remember that foreplay is about more than simply physical pleasure; it's also about connecting with your spouse. Talking, cuddling, and showing affection may improve the whole experience and make it more pleasurable for both people. Don't be hesitant to experiment with new approaches or activities to keep things interesting. Remember that the purpose of foreplay is to create arousal and anticipation, so take your time and enjoy the ride.

Oral sex abilities

Teasing Techniques to Make Her Want You More

Building anticipation is a critical component of perfecting foreplay. Teasing tactics like kissing her neck or toying with her hair might assist in enhancing tension and desire. Delaying gratification can also help to create a more intense and long-lasting experience. Alternate between soft and more intense touches, or move away from her sensitive places just as she's ready to climax. Remember, the goal is to keep her wanting more, so don't be hesitant to experiment with different ways.

1. Experiment with breast/nipple play.
Beginning with mild caressing, circling, or kissing the nipples, or softly cradling the breasts, may truly excite your lover during foreplay.

2. Nibble and/or lick the inside of the thigh

building up the suspense by nibbling or sucking the inner thigh as you begin to descend. Feel free to investigate additional places with your lips or hands, such as the neck, stomach, and buttocks.

3. Wear your underpants.

Stroke the vulva or clit while still wearing your underpants. You're creating suspense once more you might even tug their underpants to the side when you're ready to make contact.

4. Make use of your breath and tongue

Warm up the entire region by running your tongue up and down while wearing your underpants. To enhance clitoral stimulation "The clitoris is the queen,. "Always and forever. Never forget it." When in doubt, keep your concentration here and listen to your spouse as they respond to different sorts of clitoral stimulation.

5. Dance with your tongue around it.

Going slowly at first is a smart idea. To begin creating a sensation, dance your tongue over the clit or softly graze it.

6. Lick it from top to bottom or side to side.

As you lick their clit up and down or side to side, pay attention to and feel your partner's response. You should be able to determine which one they like, and it never hurts to ask!

7. **Experiment with sucking on it.**

Some enjoy it, some don't, but if they're into it, try softly sucking on the clit between strokes.

8. **Maintain consistency.**

If your partner plainly loves what you're doing, keep the movement and rhythm steady. Changing techniques or speeds often might make it difficult for them to relax into the experience.

Kiss or kiss the genitalia Don't overlook the lips! The labia (both the inner and outer sets) are also sensitive, and stimulating that area can provide a more complete experience.

9. Distribute the labia

Spread the labia apart to truly expose the clit, and your spouse will feel everything much more intensely.

10. Take a breast

Again, breasts and nipples are extremely sensitive

some people orgasm just from nipple stimulation. Reach up with your free hand and grip their breast and/or stroke their nipple as you go down on them.

11. Try inserting one or two fingers.

You can use one or two fingers to penetrate the vagina if your spouse loves to be penetrated while oral (some don't so ask!). Just don't "smash them inside ,While kissing their clit, lightly touch the G-spot with your fingers in a curling motion. Check to see whether they enjoy tongue penetration. Some individuals prefer tongue penetration when getting head, but it doesn't provide as much sensation as, say, licking the clit. See how they react, and if they like it, alternate your tongue between the clit and vagina.

12. If they're into it, play with their buttocks.

Some people love anal stimulation while receiving head, whether through their fingers or their mouth. Remember to always obtain consent, and make sure you understand their hygiene preferences. (If you're nervous, a test run in the shower is a terrific place to start; for more ideas, check out our shower sex guide.)

17. Include toys.

Sex toys aren't just for solitary enjoyment; they may also be an excellent supplement to a healthy sex life with your partner. Furthermore, the possibilities are limitless dependent on your and your partner's preferences. Consider vibrators, butt plugs, nipple clamps, or anything you're into.

18. Consider watching porn.

If you and your lover are both like movies, viewing oral sex porn might add a little more spice (and inspiration) to the encounter.

Positions for oral sex

Changing positions may be an excellent method to stimulate various places and provide varied feelings depending on how long it takes them to climax.

1. one person lying on their back and the other delivering head from the side, perpendicular to their partner's body. This posture provides a fresh perspective, additional vulva stimulation, and the opportunity to reach more sensitive areas.

2. Oral sex from the back

Give them a head from behind from a doggie stance. This posture is also ideal if your spouse enjoys rimming.

3. seated on your face

This is a popular position among many since it provides an excellent angle for the provider as well as loads of access to the rest of the receiver's body, such as gripping their breasts or buttocks. Throw out a "sit on my face" when you first start hooking up or anytime you want to shift positions to ratchet up the heat.

4. On your knees,

oral Giving head on your knees may seem more often

linked with blowjobs, but it may be hot for almost anybody. Remember to widen your labia here for greater clitoral exposure.

5. Taking oral notes Assign a chair to the receiving partner.

Bonus points if it's in an unusual location, such as the kitchen table or a living room chair. You have easy access from below since their legs are draped over the edges of the chair.

6.   The   pillow technique

Place cushions beneath their hips. Using a cushion to raise their hips forward slightly allows their legs to expand somewhat wider, exposing more of the anus.

Chapter 3

Sex positions to make her scream with delight

If you're not getting much out of sex, you're not alone, and the positions you're in might be part of the issue (or, at the very least, not part of the cure). Perhaps you're filling these roles because your partner wants you to or because you believe you should. However, this does not guarantee that your body will respond orgasmically if the posture is not intended for your enjoyment. You'll not only find the finest sex positions for female orgasms.

Why Don't You Orgasm During Sex?

Many people believe that sex occurs when a penis penetrates a vagina, and most women will not respond to this type of stimulation. Why? Most women require direct clitoral stimulation to attain orgasm, which penetration does not provide. Why do we insist on these gender roles? They're what we see or hear about, even if they're not the most obscene sex positions.

If you're coming during penetration, it might be because your clitoris is sensitive and close to your vagina. If the distance between your urethra and clit is more than the length of your thumb from the tip of your thumb to the first knuckle (approximately one inch), you are less likely to orgasm during sex . However, many women have a clitoris that is about an inch away from their vaginal entrance, thus they are simply not stimulated during sex.

Do you want to know whether you're a lucky lady with a clit-to-vag distance of less than one inch? To check, simply insert your thumb into your pantyhose. You may, however, get a little more up close and personal with a tiny hand mirror over which you can crouch to examine your anatomy.

Female Orgasm's Favorite Sex Positions

The following are only a handful of the finest orgasmic positions.

1. Cowgirl

When you're on top, you have complete control over the angle, pace, and depth of penetration. By the way, as a woman, sex positions in which you have control work best for achieving climax.

Why?

If you want to obtain the excitement you want, you must be in command. You may even reach down and touch your clit, or use a toy, and your boyfriend can assist as well. Here's a tip that can help drive you over the edge: have your partner wrap two fingers around the base of his penis on either side. While riding him, the knuckles give something to brush against.

Are you afraid of reaching the top? Don't be concerned; this is quite normal!

2. Doggy Fashion

Doggy style is an ideal posture for orgasm due to G-spot feelings rather than clitoral stimulation (advice here). If you like G Spot, then doggie could be just up your alley. Some couples find it difficult to doggy because of height issues, so consider putting a pillow beneath your legs or crouching on a piece of furniture as your boyfriend enters you from behind. Placing cushions beneath your stomach might help you keep your weight.

If you enjoy clitoral stimulation, don't worry. If you or your spouse wants to reach between your legs and assist you in the climax, Doggy allows enough access to your clit.

3. Coital Alignment Method

The Coital Alignment Technique, or CAT, was created expressly to address the lack of orgasms . This approach might assist you in having greater orgasmic experiences during sex.

In a few essential areas, CAT varies from Missionary. One, your boyfriend should get closer to you than he normally would in missionary mode. Then, raise your hips so your clitoris is closer to your partner's pelvis (a cushion under your buttocks helps). This allows you to grind him down. Then, instead of pushing, he concentrates on a rocking motion.

4. Lotus

This sex position may not suit every body shape and size, but it's worth a go if you believe it may. To enter the Lotus sex position, have your boyfriend sit down and cross his legs like a pretzel. You then sit in his lap, your legs wrapped over his back. If you like, you can lock your ankles behind him.

Because of the face-to-face contact and the opportunity to kiss, the position is extremely personal. You'll also notice that rocking works better than thrusting in this position, which is why it's one of her finest.

5. The Thigh Tide

This is a Reverse Cowgirl version that makes use of grinding. All you have to do is have your spouse bend one knee and place his foot flat on the bed. This brings his thigh forward in front of you. You may grind against it while rocking your hips and maintain the same control as in the Cowgirl position.

You may wrap your arms over his knee for extra support if you like.

6. Rear Entrance

You might not believe this is one of the finest places to orgasm, but hear us out. Although lying on your stomach as your spouse enters you from behind is an easy sex position, you may modify it for superb clitoral stimulation.

To begin, place a cushion beneath your hips to grind against. If you prefer firmness, narrow pillows are ideal. Alternatively, use a softer pillow to elevate your hips and insert your favorite vibrator between your body and the pillow. Some sex pillows even have openings where you can insert vibrators while using them!

7. Missionary

Okay, we've explored how, while the Missionary position isn't always one of the finest sex positions for women, it may get you to the climax you deserve if done correctly. To begin, play with your clit or encourage your man to do so if there is adequate space between your bodies. Second, you may keep a tiny vibrator that curves against your body between the two of you while having sex.

How to Have Orgasm Through Sex

Aside from trying out some of the finest sex positions for female orgasms, you can utilize some of the following tips to get the most out of your bedroom escapades.

Make use of toys.

Toys make orgasming simpler or are essential for certain ladies. Toys may last longer than your hand or partner, as long as the batteries are charged. It also relieves your spouse of the pressure of maintaining an erection.

Concentrate on more than simply penile penetration.

Sure, PIV sex normally works for guys, but it doesn't work for many women. It doesn't imply you can't have orgasm, just not with penetration. Incorporate his or her fingers and tongues to ensure climax throughout sex. Even a carefully positioned thigh might provide you with orgasmic pleasure.

Grind it out. Grinding and humping are excellent methods to stimulate your clitoris, but many sex positions do not allow for this. The finest sex positions for women may be ones that allow you to grind against your partner's body while he's within you. Another possibility is to grind against a cushion.

Make use of pillows.

Pillows aren't simply for sleeping.

Suitable for humping. They might make it simpler to enter into or stay in certain positions until you can orgasm. Stiffer pillows are better for placement, and manufacturers like Liberator provide memory foam pillows designed expressly for sex.

Apply lubricant.

Lube facilitates initial penetration while also allowing you to go further. So, lubrication is your buddy if you're a lady who needs a little extra time to get off (and there's nothing wrong with that!)

Don't forget about foreplay.

The more excited you are before your boyfriend even gets between your legs, the more probable an orgasm will occur during penetration.

with your sexual partner all work together to create the tone for your sex life.

Whether you're having sex with a devoted partner, a casual fling, or anywhere in between, the relationship between you two is undeniably important in how much you get out of your sex life. Many factors contribute to that dynamic, including your expectations for each other and the relationship, how much you enjoy each other's presence, and, most importantly, trust.

Trust and sexual pleasure are inextricably linked.

This may seem simple, but there's a lot more to the term "trust" than meets the eye. So, how does trust manifest itself in our sexual life, and how can it be increased within a relationship? Let us investigate!

Using 'Trustworthy' to Your Advantage

When used appropriately, trust and the perception of being trustworthy may be your hidden weapon and biggest advantage.

Are you seeking a soulmate relationship? If so, you're seeking a mature woman. She has moved on from the Tinder phase of her dating life and is searching for true, stable, long-term love. This woman seeks a man who exemplifies dependability.

If you want to become more appealing to her, she must regard you as trustworthy.

A man who exudes trust is 10 times more appealing to a woman.

Women are biologically predisposed to prefer guys they believe to be trustworthy.

And, according to natural factors, they are seeking a long-term companion. Having a reliable long-term spouse, biologically speaking, ensures that their progeny will have food, shelter, and safety.
This is the primary reason why a woman seeks a trustworthy spouse. She's on the lookout for someone who can satisfy her subconscious (or conscious!) desire for security.

A reliable man makes a lady feel safe and open.

She is at ease and can relax into the connection with confidence. When a woman feels protected, the metaphorical chains fall away, allowing her to fully express her femininity and feminine nature.

This will heighten the polarity and make her more alluring to you. If trust is the glue that holds a relationship together, polarity is the magnet that attracts a man and a woman in the first place.

To Become Trustworthy, Work On Trust.

As previously said, the cause for being labeled 'untrustworthy' is frequently intimately linked with our own lack of trust in the world around us and in ourselves. Working on your capacity to trust yourself and others is therefore the first step in becoming more trustworthy to women and having the relationship of your dreams.

A mature guy trusts. He is sturdy, dependable, and trustworthy. He is totally expressing his divine manhood and acting in accordance with his higher nature.

Understanding Sex And Trust

What comes to mind when you think of the word "trust" in the context of relationships? Keeping promises? Being able to trust someone? What about physical and mental security? All of these are essential components of interpersonal trust, but there's a lot more to the tale.

Trust is more than just being able to rely on someone. On a deeper level, trust is the subtle capacity to be really present with someone. When you have a high degree of trust in someone, you may bring your whole self to the table. Trust helps you to feel comfortable with your spouse; a distinct degree of relaxation adds to pleasure and happiness.

If you don't entirely trust your sexual partner, it doesn't necessarily indicate that they are "untrustworthy," but that you don't feel comfortable completely opening up to them on some level. That doesn't imply one of you is at fault, but rather that something in the relationship is wrong.

When your sex life isn't fulfilling your expectations, it's tempting to blame your spouse or yourself, but it's no one's responsibility. If you're having difficulty developing deep trust in a sexual or romantic relationship, it might be due to unresolved traumas from any age. These incidents cause a disruption in your capacity to connect with people on the level you desire, particularly in sexual or romantic interactions. A lack of trust is frequently caused by internal issues that manifest themselves in your relationship and, of course, your sex life.

It takes time to build trust.

Even if you're confident in yourself, trust doesn't happen overnight. It takes time to develop the amount of trust that is typically required for you to have the type of pleasure that you desire. When you devote time to nurturing this aspect of your relationship, it begins to foster a sense of safety and security. This, in turn, helps you to totally open up to this individual in every way.

It takes time to establish sexual pleasure through foreplay, kissing, and sensuous touch. However, it also has to do with the larger picture of establishing trust and enjoyment in the partnership as a whole. You may want to rush through and enjoy everything right now, but certain things are worth the wait. However, there are several things you can do to assist in creating the type of trust that allows for more closeness and pleasure.

How to Increase Trust in Relationships

Trust develops intuitively in relationships, but it may also be developed via deliberate activity.

Here are some strategies for increasing trust in your relationship:

Honesty is more than simply not lying. Being honest is being open about your expectations, wants, and desires in the relationship. It expresses what's in your thoughts and in your heart.

Pleasure and joy are inextricably linked. Positive experiences contribute to the development of trust. Consider methods to offer greater joy to the relationship, such as sharing mutual interests, dancing or cooking together, or anything!

Because trust frequently boils down to you, you may need to undertake some self-healing work on yourself, which will then ripple out into your relationship.

In Healthy Sex, trust is a crucial attribute. It makes us feel emotionally comfortable and confident in our decision to continue being in an intimate connection with our spouse. Without trust, we are more prone to experience worry, dread, disappointment, and betrayal.

When both persons in a partnership perform appropriately and follow through on agreements, trust increases. While no one can promise that a relationship will endure and be pleasant for both parties, you may improve mutual trust by establishing clear expectations of each other in the relationship.

Spend time with your spouse talking about what you need and expect from your relationship in order to feel emotionally safe. Create a list of understandings that you will both agree to honor based on your talk. You could wish to codify your list into a "contract" that you will adhere to. An example of a Healthy

Sex trust contract is shown below. These shared understandings are frequently helpful in creating trust in a healthy sexual relationship. Use this sample list to assist you and your spouse in developing your own set of relationship ground rules.

set of relationship ground rules.

We all agree on the following:

It is OK to refuse sex AT ANY TIME.

It is OK to ask for what we want sexually without being mocked or chastised for doing so.

We are never forced to do something sexual that we do not want to do.

We shall take a pause or discontinue sexual activity if any of us asks for it.

It is OK to express how we are feeling or what we require AT ANY TIME.

We pledge to be sensitive to each other's bodily comfort requirements.

What we do sexually is private and should not be mentioned with anybody outside of our relationship unless we give consent. We are ultimately accountable for our own sexual satisfaction and orgasm. Our sexual dreams and thoughts are our own, and we don't have to share them with one another unless we want to. We are not required to divulge the specifics of a former sexual connection unless it is critical to our current partner's physical health or safety.

We can initiate or deny sex without our partner reacting negatively.

We each promise to be sexually monogamous unless we have a clear, previous agreement that having sex outside the partnership is acceptable (this includes virtual sex, such as phone or internet sex).

We will work together to reduce risk and use protection to reduce the potential of illness and/or undesired pregnancy.

We both agree to be checked for sexually transmitted diseases at any time.

We shall promptly tell each other if we have or think we have a sexually transmitted infection.

If we believe or know that a pregnancy has resulted from our lovemaking, we shall notify each other.

We shall help each other in dealing with any bad results of our lovemaking.

Chapter 4

How to Last Longer and Remain Harder in her clitoris

We don't need to remember that your penis doesn't always operate as it should. You undoubtedly discovered throughout puberty that you occasionally experience erections at inconvenient times. As you get older, you may discover that the opposite is also true, it might be difficult to get and stay hard when you want to. Erection issues can make you feel as if your body is actively conspiring against you. You can't seem to get it up with your lover when things get hot and heavy. Things go wild down there after a few swallows of wine. You struggle in the bedroom after a tough day at work. Feeling out of control of your own body, especially when it comes to sex, maybe unpleasant and embarrassing. You may believe that your erection problems are a reflection of your sexual ability (which is incorrect), and your partner may believe that it is their fault that you aren't getting hard (which is also incorrect). It's no surprise that erectile dysfunction is frequently related to stress and worry. But don't worry; neither you nor your partner are to blame.

Poor erections are often caused by one of five factors:

(reduced blood flow, aberrant hormone levels, medication, improper nerve activity, and the mental component). Making lifestyle and nutritional modifications, as well as speaking with sexual partners, may all help a person get stronger erections. To discover the optimal answer, people should collaborate with healthcare specialists.

Persistent erectile dysfunction may be an indication of an underlying psychological or physical disorder in certain circumstances. Certain drugs might also make it difficult to obtain and sustain an erection. This post will look at several alternatives for improving erectile function and when you should consult a doctor.

What exactly is erectile dysfunction?

Erectile dysfunction (ED) refers to difficulties obtaining or maintaining an erection. ED is a common, generally curable disorder in which a person is unable to obtain or maintain an erection long enough for sexual engagement. It most commonly affects men over the age of 40, but it can occur at any age. Some people with ED may be able to achieve an erection, but it may not stay long enough for intercourse, and they may not be able to have an erection every time they want to have sex.

Others may be unable to develop an erection at all.

What causes erection difficulties?

1. Consult with your partner.

Struggling to get up and stay up might contribute to performance anxiety in the bedroom, especially if you're attempting to please a new person. When the time comes to get down, you may get so concerned about not getting down that you, well, don't get down.

" Say something like, 'Just a heads up; I sometimes get in my head and struggle with getting hard.'" Before you have sex, discuss your erection troubles with your partner and tell them it has nothing to do with your desire for them. I simply want you to understand that it has nothing to do with you. "I find you very hot; I just get a bit worried every now and again." "Odds are, your lover will appreciate your candor and vulnerability.

2. Consult a physician.

If a person is having difficulty obtaining or keeping an erection, they should consult a doctor. They can talk about potential reasons, do testing, and, if required, prescribe medicine. Check your testosterone levels. Low testosterone does not directly impair the mechanics involved in your erection, but it does affect your desire, making it more difficult to turn on and more difficult to become, well, hard.

Whether you experience an unusual decline in your sex drive or any of these signs of low testosterone, you should consult your doctor to see whether your T levels are low. If they are, your doctor can help you restore your testosterone levels back to normal. Seeking therapy may also help prevent possible EDTrusted Source problems, such as a lack of pleasure in their sex lives. relationship infidelity, sadness, anxiety, and poor self-esteem issues conceiving

3. Consume a well-balanced diet.

A diet that promotes heart health may also promote penile health. eating a Mediterranean diet may help sustain erectile function. Obesity and high blood pressure, which are risk factors for heart disease, can also raise the likelihood of erectile dysfunction. Adopting a Mediterranean diet may aid in the reduction of cardiovascular risk factors.

A Mediterranean diet consists of the following foods:
A variety of fruits and vegetables, nuts, whole grains legumes, including lentils, peas, and beans a moderate amount of fish and a moderate amount of alcohol, such as a glass of wine with dinner. a low dairy and meat intake a low candy intake exercises are performed. "Contractions of the pelvic floor muscles help produce an increase in penis pressure and rigidity of the penis. exercises, which include contracting and relaxing your

pelvic floor muscles, can help strengthen your erections.

4. A lot of yawns.

Sorry if simply reading the word "yawn" made you yawn. Actually, we're not sorry because yawning and getting an erection is the same thing in your body. Nitric oxide, a chemical, regulates both of them. When it is released in the brain, it can either travel to the neurons that regulate mouth opening and breathing, or it can travel down the spinal cord to the blood vessels that supply the penis. Sometimes it does both .

Her orgasm

Orgasm is a bodily response that happens when the pelvic floor muscles contract and relax in a repetitive pattern. Orgasms have emotional implications in addition to offering physical relief. During an orgasm, often known as a climax, your body produces feel-good hormones such as oxytocin.

1 The oxytocin released during an orgasm, as well as the skin-to-skin contact during sex, aid in emotional bonding with your partner.

Pap, Eat and struck her erogenous zone for her orgasm.

- **Orgasmic Nipple Orgasm**

Because your breasts and nipples are important erogenous zones, stimulating those areas might result in an orgasm. Because they contain so many nerve endings, the nipples are highly sensitive to touch. There is no apparent agreement on how many women can orgasm without touching their genitals. However, studies have shown that nipple stimulation triggers the region of your brain that regulates genital sensation.

- **Orgasmic Clitoral Orgasm**
The clitoris is a sexual organ that appears as a little erect tissue on the vulva's outside but extends inside into your vagina. It is composed of millions of nerve endings, making it extremely responsive to stimuli.

- **Directly stimulating the clitoris or**

caressing the labia surrounding the clitoris
increases blood flow to the region, causing the clitoris to become engorged and in need of orgasmic release.

- **Orgasm on the G-Spot**
Though research is mixed, the general agreement on the G-spot is that it is positioned in the front wall of your vagina, approximately halfway between your vaginal

entrance and cervix. Some experts believe it's a sex organ, while others feel it's part of the clitoris' nerve-ending network. Some people claim that a G-spot orgasm is far more powerful than other forms of orgasms.

• Orgasm in the cervix

A vaginal orgasm is defined as an orgasm caused by penetrative vaginal intercourse that does not purposely stimulate the clitoris and

G-spot. The vagina possesses extra erogenous zones in addition to the clitoris. The A-spot, also known as the anterior fornix, is found on the vagina's high front (or anterior) wall, immediately beneath the cervix. When handled correctly, this region can cause a profound vaginal orgasm. Touching the cervix may also cause orgasm in certain people. This is due to the presence of ligaments with nerves that might be extremely sensitive in certain locations.

Several orgasms for her Multiple orgasms are like unicorns in the sex world.

Women who can have them feel immense pleasure, but those who haven't fully mastered the technique are sometimes suspicious that it's even possible. Fortunately, you may be able to develop this ability, and we have some pointers for you. What precisely is a multiple orgasm? It is dependent on the woman. It might entail having numerous orgasms in a single session or being able to attain orgasms rapidly. For example, if you can have more than one orgasm in a five- or ten-minute period, you

would consider yourself
multi-orgasmic. These are
also known as consecutive
orgasms. He deserves an
orgasm.

Chapter 5

The penetrating act

Ahhh... those initial frantic seconds when the penis meets the labia. When every sexual sensory cell in your body craves to be touched. When the thrill of conquering is about to be repaid. There is an art to enhancing these emotions of penetration for you and your lover and you are the artist.

Knowing she would feel these initial few seconds of bliss differently than you is critical to making your masterpiece. What is it that she desires? How can it be boosted? Come investigate and find out. But, before you start exploring, there are a few things you should do to ensure maximum enjoyment for both you and your partner:

Lubricate Your Relationship

It undoubtedly goes against every bone in your body, especially that huge throbbing one, but unless your girlfriend expresses a desire for it hard and fast right away, resist the urge to push. Why? She isn't prepared.

If you try to penetrate your sweetheart before she's properly warmed, she won't feel very loving. It's rude, and selfish, and can make her uncomfortable or even painful. Keep in mind that if she's dry, you should be ready. You're good to go if she's moist.

Grab a bottle of Slippery Lube and smear it on your sweetheart to get her ready for the trip.

Give Her an Exotic Labial Massage.

This massage isn't on any spa's menu, but add it to yours and she'll flow like a fountain.

Pour some sex lubricant or saliva right into the action and distribute it about so you're both gleaming and slick.

Slowly move the head of your slick erect penis up to the entrance of her vagina with your hand. Refrain from going too deep! Instead, gradually tease by circling the tip all the way around the hole, then gliding it between her labia up to her clitoris. Slide it back down to the entrance after a few enticing clitoral swirls.

Repeat your seductive laps up and down her labia with many more sensual laps. Admire the scenery, appreciate the feelings, take your time, and use all of your talents to stay outside. Your rewards will arrive soon.

Making Your Big Debut

When you can't take it any longer, slip the head of your penis inside with your hand. Feel her soft lips embrace you as you trigger the millions of pleasure cells in her vaginal mouth.

But now isn't the moment to go on autopilot; instead, utilize your sixth sense to match the angle of your erection to her acceptance angle. Begin cautiously, and if everything is in order, move a bit deeper, then deeper, then deeper, until you're entirely within.

Many women refer to this as the "hurts so good" moment when your massive penetration and the exhilarating sensation of fullness stretch the vagina wider with pleasure. If your partner is expressive, her passionate vocalizations will reveal it.

You now have a decision to make. You can start hammering in-out or you can wow her with some amazing sensuous powers, which is just what she wants!

Turn On Your Pump

By definition, the male has some (or all) control over the pumping. So, why limit yourself to only driving in one gear?

Heads up, Bob.

To entice her, stroke shallowly, in-out, using only the head of your penis for a bit, nothing deeper.

Platter with many options.
 Try three mini-pumps a few inches within, then one long, deep, beautiful push. Repeat in a rhythmic manner.
Grind of the Gods.

 Show her you know her by slowly...sensually...erotically... grinding your soft pubic bone against her fragile clitoris...while your penis enters her.

Knead to get up to speed.

Accelerate your pumping toward climax after a slow, enticing start. If you feel like you're approaching too quickly, downshift and try the Divine Grind.

The Dangle is angled.

Your aim is to locate ALL of your lover's interior pleasure regions. Pivot and curve your penis all around her till she moves and moans in delight.

I adore Lever G.

Angle and place your penis within for precise G-spot rubbing.

Hot-hammer.

Some ladies enjoy it quickly and hard. Some people don't know unless they try it. And the rest will despise it. So give it a shot and if she squeals with excitement, keep drilling!

The Rhythm Nation.

It's the rhythm that makes sex known as horizontal dance. Pump to the exhilaration of making love together, pounding, grinding, and gyrating in tune with your shared passion as your entire body swings in accord, including hips, shoulders, and knees.

Whether this is your first time or a refresher course, the greatest joys of sex are now in your skilled hands!

Sexual analgesia (Anal sex)

What is anal sex and how is it performed? Are there any dangers?

Anal intercourse occurs when a penis or other item is placed into the anus of a partner. Like any other sexual action, some people enjoy it while others do not. Some individuals are intrigued by it, while others are aware that it is not something they are comfortable with. There is nothing wrong with having anal intercourse, but only you can determine whether it is suitable for you.

Because the anus cannot produce its own lubrication (like the vagina can) and the tissue of the anus is particularly delicate, it is critical that extra water-soluble lubricant should be used during anal intercourse. Without lubrication, the anus may experience pain, discomfort, and tissue tears. As with any other sort of intercourse, comfort and relaxation are essential for a good experience during anal intercourse. Slowly push a penis into the anus and stop if there is discomfort or resistance. It's better if a person poops before anal intercourse and washes thoroughly before and after anal sex or oral-anal contact. Couples who participate in anal intercourse should be aware that it is one of the ways STIs/HIV may be transmitted sexually. This is because the anus lining is prone to ripping if there is little lubrication. This causes tiny rips in the anus, making it easier for STIs, including HIV, to enter. Safer sex, like any other sort of sex, is important during anal intercourse. There are several strategies to lower the risk of acquiring or transmitting a sexually transmitted infection (STI) during anal intercourse. If you're conducting anal penetration with your finger, for example, you can use a condom on the penis. You can also place an internal (female) condom into the anus using an internal (female) condom on the penis. You can apply a dental dam over the anal region to prevent oral-anal contact.

People have a wide range of emotions when it comes to anal intercourse. Some individuals believe that only homosexual people have anal sex. But that is not the case. People of all sexual orientations can and do engage in anal intercourse. At the same time, some couples avoid anal intercourse.

When having anal intercourse, never put the penis into the vagina after it has been in the anus without first replacing the condom or cleaning the penis. Anus bacteria can cause serious vaginal infections. Furthermore, regardless of each partner's sex, after the penis has been in a partner's anus, it should never be entered into a partner's mouth without first replacing the condom or cleaning the penis. Bacteria in the anus can cause serious vaginal infections, as well as oral and intestinal illnesses. It is also possible to become pregnant from anal intercourse if semen flows from the anus into the vaginal entrance, which is not far away yet another reason to use a condom.

Make sure you and your partner have talked and agreed on anal intercourse before indulging in it.

How does anal function?

When having anal sex, two things are critical: **take it gently and use enough lube.**

Unlike the vagina, the anus lacks natural lubrication. However, if you want anal intercourse to be painless, you will need to compensate with plenty of lubrication.

In addition, your partner must be very calm so that the muscles around the anus are not tense. You should begin by caressing the anus, and then after a time, you may insert a finger and watch how your spouse reacts. If everything is in order, you can insert the head of your penis.

Move at a glacial pace.
Rapid motions will cause pain.
Anal sex takes some getting
used to, and the slower you
move and the more time and
lubrication you use, the more
likely you are to like it!

Is Anal filthy?

Before havinganal
intercourse, ask your spouse to
go to the bathroom and cleanse
the region around the anus

with soapy water. However, enemas are not required (in fact, they can irritate the anus and bowel).

The rectum is the 'tube' inside your anus. It serves as a holding area for feces that is about to exit the body. If you're healthy and don't have diarrhea, constipation, or intestinal illnesses, the rectum is left empty and relatively clean until the next batch of waste arrives.

If you're concerned about becoming dirty but still desire anal sex, start in the shower.

Remember that water-based lubricant will wash away in the shower, so use silicone-based lubrication instead.

What is the source of this pleasant sensation?

Men enjoy anal sex because their prostate receives a lot of attention. The prostate is a walnut-sized gland that may be felt approximately five cm within the rectum through the

wall. Stimulating the prostate may produce very fantastic orgasms in a man.
Furthermore, the anus and rectum are significantly tighter than the vagina, making insertion particularly enjoyable for males.

Women like anal intercourse because the anus has numerous nerve endings, making it incredibly sensitive to touch (men, too, have such nerve endings). Stimulation feels wonderful and can be really pleasurable.

STDs and anal sex

When you have anal intercourse, you are at a significant risk of contracting an STD. Because the anus lacks natural lubrication, it is quite possible that tiny tears may form surrounding it during anal intercourse. This makes it incredibly simple for viruses such as HIV to enter your body. That is why, when having anal intercourse, you should always use a condom!

Also, don't proceed from the anus to the vagina without first washing the penis (finger or toy) and replacing the condom - the bacteria that live around the anus can cause vaginal infections.

Anal is not homosexual.

Some people believe that anal intercourse is reserved for

homosexuals. This is not correct. Anyone can engage in anal sex. To begin with, homosexual sex isn't exclusively anal. And not all homosexual men are interested. According to one survey, somewhat more than 50% of homosexual males have anal intercourse on a regular basis.

When men learn they love anal action, they may question their sexual orientation. However, due to the tremendous sensations and orgasms individuals can have from having their prostate massaged, they shouldn't be too concerned. Don't be hesitant if you're straight: if you want your lover to put a finger inside, talk to her or show her.

Sexual desires

Sexual fancies are very natural. Some of them may appear strange, but just because you fantasize about something does not obligate you to perform it.

Fantasy is typical.

The majority of individuals have fantasies. Sexual fantasies are images or thoughts in your brain that make you feel hot. They might be your ideas or memories of anything you've seen, read, or experienced, such as a pornographic film or a hot night with someone. Fantasies do not have to be openly sexual; what arouses you is entirely personal. Some individuals are attracted to tunnels because they are reminiscent of vaginas. Nothing is weird when it comes to fantasy!

Because fantasies are created by your mind, they might include concepts that would be considered bad, odd, forbidden, or even criminal in real life.
If you believe your imagination is particularly bizarre or unusual, don't panic;

chances are, it's not at all unusual.

Only when fantasies entail activities on non-consenting people do they become problematic. Doctors then label the delusion as "pathological," regardless of whether it is acted on.

Because it might be difficult to discuss sex and sexual fantasies in real life, some psychologists believe that fantasies provide a means for the "brain to go wild," picturing things that would otherwise go unspoken in real life. Even if you'd never ask your spouse to explore BDSM, you may indulge your kinky fantasies in your thoughts.

Fantasy does not have to become a reality.

Almost everyone has sexual fantasies, but only a small percentage of people act on them. Even if you fantasize about something like a threesome, you probably wouldn't want to do it in real life.

That's why you shouldn't be too concerned about your dreams - just because you're straight and fantasize about having sex with someone of the same gender doesn't indicate you're homo- or bisexual. Similarly, fantasizing about having sex with someone other than your partner should not be interpreted as a desire to cheat. You should not feel ashamed or guilty about your fantasies;

instead, consider them a healthy approach for your brain to explore unexplored aspects of sexuality with some interest.

Although both sexes have sexual fantasies, research suggests that women are less likely to wish to act on them. Aside from that, the imaginations of the different genders are pretty similar.

Popular delusions

So, what are some of the fancies that individuals have?

This is only a partial list; there are many, many more.

Threesomes for oral sex

Being seen or videotaped
Observing other individuals
Being exposed in public
Sexual activity in public places
Sex with complete strangers
Sex in groups
Sex with someone who is extremely

large/small/tall/skinny/older, and so on.

Sex with another person of the same gender

Having sex with celebs

Sexual analgesia

Putting your fantasies into action

Sharing some of your desires with your spouse may be exciting and energizing. You may even try to act out some of the pictures your brain came up with if you want to and they agree.

If you're uncomfortable bringing it up, try lightly addressing it, such as by stating you've read about sex in public places. Assess your partner's reaction and, if they are interested, ask if it is something the two of you can pursue.

Acting out fantasies through role-playing is a widespread practice. For example, if you had a dream about having sex with a stranger, your partner might act as someone you don't know. You can meet at a pub and talk to each other as if you've never met before. Then you may take them to a hotel room or your house for a one-night stand.

But don't be dismayed if things don't go exactly as planned; the brain is a great tool that can sometimes make things appear better than they are.

Conclusion

Understanding female anatomy, the science of arousal, and techniques like commutation, kissing, and sensual touches can help guys provide a more satisfying and fulfilling experience for their woman. Remember to pay attention to hygiene and grooming to avoid common mistakes and be open to trying new things always.

With foreplay practice, you may develop a deeper, more pleasant connection with your woman.

www.ingramcontent.com/pod-product-compliance
Lightning Source LLC
Chambersburg PA
CBHW070927260726
48661CB00003B/846